SO YOU WANT TO EAT HEALTHIER

CASSIE LEIGH

ALSO BY CASSIE LEIGH

Quick & Easy Cooking for One

TABLE OF CONTENTS

INTRODUCTION

What am I doing writing a book about being healthier? I don't know, but here we are.

Recently I had to lose 10% of my body weight for health reasons, which had me thinking about eating healthy and losing weight and sustainable weight loss. And about how hard it is to "eat healthy" when what that means for every single person is different.

For me, for example, eating heart-healthy might mean eating something like spinach. For someone who has had open-heart surgery and is on life-long blood thinners, spinach would be a horrible idea, because it would mess with the effectiveness of their medications.

Another example. I remember growing up when everyone was into eating grapefruit for breakfast, because *that* was supposedly healthy for you. But many medicines that people take these days don't mix well with grapefruit, which means it isn't for them.

So eating healthy has to be a personal thing because only you know your situation.

There's also the psychology of it. I know a woman who has been a health nut forever. One of the things she eats for breakfast is an egg white omelet with salsa. Sounds healthy, right? I also had a co-worker who used to snack on soy nuts. Also healthy.

Which, hey, if you can eat tasteless food and be satisfied, that's great. But for most of us, that's not going to be the case, and trying to force ourselves to eat flavorless "healthy" foods is going to backfire. Because we won't be able to sustain that year in and year out for the rest of our lives. For a couple weeks for a vacation or a couple months for a wedding? Sure. But for a lifetime? Hell no.

So instead of giving you specific recipes or a diet to follow, I'm going to spend this book talking about healthy eating in general as well as mental attitude, lifestyle, and personal philosophy. Those are the areas you have to really master to lose weight *and keep it off long-term.*

Now, I'm not a nutrition expert. I'm not a doctor. I'm also not some uber-healthy marathon runner. I'm just a person who was in the overweight category, who needed to bring that down, and has some healthy, sustainable (hopefully) tricks for doing so.

Maybe they will work for you, maybe they won't. Maybe they help you find what does work for you even if it wouldn't work for me. (Soy nuts anyone?)

Even if you don't manage to lose a bunch of weight (which is probably, honestly, not a good idea if you want to keep what you lose off), I want you to walk away from this book healthier. Or with a plan for how to be healthier.

I was going to include recipes in this book, but honestly there are recipes available everywhere for free. Better to give you the foundation to build on than "the answer", which doesn't actually exist and is different for each person.

Introduction

So you're going to have to take those next steps yourself, keeping in mind what will work best *for you* and your health issues.

Okay then, let's get started.

HOW I HAVE LOST WEIGHT

I have lost 10% or more of my body weight three times in my life.

The first was when I was broke as could be and went back to college. I was suddenly walking all over a large campus every day (so exercising more) while living on one-dollar muffins and fast food apple pies (so eating less).

I did not intend to lose weight, but the combination of not enough calories and lots of additional exercise made me drop a significant amount of weight in just four months.

Not a recommended approach, as we'll discuss later.

The second time was a deliberate attempt to lose weight. I was hiking an hour or two every day at the time and I decided I would also count calories. I researched what a good calorie level was for me given my height, and then I tracked every single thing I ate or drank, and didn't allow myself above X calories per day.

It worked. I lost that weight. But it was not healthy for me mentally. Tracking everything I ate and obsessing about calories like that set up a very unhealthy relationship with my food. One that I could see had the potential to lead to bad places. So I stopped. And eventually gained that weight back.

I actually gained it back the first time, too, because when I realized I'd dropped that weight unintentionally, I deliberately started eating big fatty burritos at least once a week. I scared myself with that weight loss. I've always prided myself that even through the worst times I still fuel my body, but I wasn't and that was bad.

The second time I lost weight I started to gain it back some when I loosened control but also because I was no longer exercising the way I had been, and I took on a stressful job assignment that I coped with by indulging my worst food habits. I'd buy a chocolate shake at lunch every day and drink beer and soda the rest of the time because I hated that assignment and did not want to be where I was.

Which brings me to this third round of weight loss. This one was prompted by a health scare. Basically, thirty-plus years of drinking soda daily finally made itself known in my liver. Not irreversibly, fortunately. I could've continued as I was, no one told me I had to stop, but I didn't want to make the damage permanent, so I chose to use this scare as a permanent wake-up call to be healthier like I've always known I should be.

My motivation is to avoid the potential of developing a chronic illness, it has nothing to do with looking good for others. (This will sound weird to some, and we'll discuss this more later, but I actually prefer to be slightly overweight. Given my druthers I would not have lost as much as I have.)

But basically this health issue came up and my doctor said the best way to treat it was to lose 10% of my body weight and, obviously, keep it off. Which meant I had to figure out a way to do so that I could stick with for the next fifty years. Egg white omelets and soy nuts were not going to work for me.

Neither were crash diets, extreme diets, or cleanses. Those are temporary fixes that your mind and body fight against. You want to look good at a wedding, you can do one of those, but don't expect it will last. (And, honestly, be careful there, too, because you can do bad things to yourself in a very short period of time by going to extremes.)

So. I knew I had to make permanent changes, which meant looking at my life and figuring out where and what I could improve *and maintain.*

There were a number of areas to consider when deciding how to make those changes. The first was my environment.

Environment

Environment and lifestyle are key parts of weight and health. If you don't have a good environment and lifestyle then you can only do so much with your weight and health.

My main issue is that I have a sweet tooth. (Likely because my mother fed me pure cane syrup in water when I was a baby when she got too tired of nursing me. True story.)

For thirty-plus years I drank multiple cans of soda a day. Most of that time it was the real-deal, full-sugar, full-caffeine version, too. I'd also eat chocolates, cake, cookies, etc. I like dessert. And to snack.

The nice part of that, is that I had an obvious target: all the sugary extras in my life.

The bad part of that is that I had a lifetime of habits built around consuming sugar. Thirsty, go to the fridge and grab a can of soda. Hungry, open that bag of chocolates.

Now, I'm lucky. I largely work from home, live alone, and don't do a lot of social activities, which means that I am in a controlled environment. If I can keep those things that are my weakness out of my home, I can eat healthy.

Fortunately, I am also lazy and cheap. This is very important, believe it or not, because it means that it takes a much larger failure of will before I will order takeout or delivery to satisfy a sugar craving.

So in my case, the first step to eating healthier was to not buy the bad things. If I could go to the store and not buy that case of soda, not buy that bag of chocolate caramel truffles, not buy that cake mix, not buy that ice cream, etc. then that was 90% of eating healthier for me.

I go to the store once a week, and as long as I resist and force myself to shop healthy for that thirty minutes, I can eat healthy for the week.

Not everyone will have that option, though. If you have to go to an office every day, or if you have kids at home, or a partner who eats unhealthy, that's going to make it much harder. So you have to look at your own environment and figure out where the weaknesses are, and then shore them up as best you can.

Maybe that means bringing lunch from home every day so you don't have to be tempted by a fast food or restaurant menu. Maybe that means that the biggest challenge to eating healthy for you is getting your partner and kids on board.

Remove as many temptation decision points as you can. And know that the more of them there are in your life, the harder it's going to be to change or to maintain that change.

Okay, so for me, a huge part of eating healthier is not bringing the bad stuff into my home. But that's just step one.

Substitutes

The next thing I did is acknowledged that I am a creature of habit. I have things I'm used to doing.

For example, I like to eat something sweet after dinner. Before I had to lose this weight it would be a small bowl of ice cream. Or coffee cake. Or maybe cookies if I'd made some.

Trying to eliminate that after dinner habit at the same time that I was trying to change what I eat, would have been too hard. So instead I substituted. I was used to having something sweet after dinner, so I continued that, but I made it healthier.

Turns out an apple is something sweet. So are berries on top of yogurt with a little drizzle of honey. Or a handful of dark chocolate chips, which, yes, are still chocolate, but they're not sugary in the same way that milk chocolate chips are. They don't leave that aftertaste of sugar on your tongue that leads to wanting more.

You have to be careful, though, and acknowledge what you will and won't do. For example, another place where I needed a substitute was soda. Based on past experience, I know that sweetened mint tea is a great substitute for cola. It has that same back of the throat feel that I like.

But turns out, as I mentioned before, I'm also lazy. Too lazy to remember to brew a new pitcher of tea every few days. So drinking cold mint tea is a hard habit for me to form, because it only lasts for a day or two before I'm standing there at the fridge thinking about how I have nothing to drink.

So this time, I straight-up switched to water. I can walk to the fridge, pour water from a pitcher into my glass, and I'm good to go. No failing at my "diet" by giving myself one of those temptation points.

(Also, that took those calories away, which is one way to lose weight. Years ago I had to give up soda for a month as part of a psychology experiment. I substituted in fruit juice instead, thinking that was healthier, but it wasn't. Fruit juice is just as high in calories and sugar.)

The other thing I had to confront is that caffeine is addictive, so I couldn't just drop soda without consequences. I now take a caffeine pill every morning to make up for that loss. Because eating healthier is hard enough without dealing with the headache that can come from caffeine withdrawal.

Habits

The third area I looked at is what habits I could develop or leverage.

I fortunately am a person who can eat the same thing day in and day out. And had been doing so for years. Last year my lunch was three slices of lunch meat with three slices of cheese, a handful of carrots, and some sort of chip.

I don't like to think at lunch time or breakfast about what I'm going to eat. Which meant that all I had to do to eat healthier is change that routine meal to something that's better for me. Lunch is now a bowl with black beans seasoned with cumin, a fried egg, salsa, and Greek yogurt. That added more fiber with the beans and took away the processed meat.

My breakfast is currently a yogurt, berries, and oats mixture that gives me a solid base to start my day alongside whole wheat bread with peanut butter. I can make the yogurt and berries mixture up and eat it every morning without thought for four days straight.

Right there, by making those meals the same every day, I ensure that two of my three meals each day are healthy for me.

Dinner is where I mix things up. But I still try to keep that to a smaller group of options that are generally healthy. Right now I'm on a big stir fry kick which involves cooking a lot of vegetables in a wok with a fish, usually salmon or tuna.

The less you have to think about what you're eating, the better, because the fewer temptation points that puts in your day. As long as the things you eat routinely are good for you, of course.

But what I do would never work for some people. I know someone who absolutely refuses to eat the same meal day after day. That person needs variety. And not just "one flavor of yogurt one day, another the next". They need complete change.

So you have to know yourself. You have to know if variety helps or hurts. And if routine helps or hurts. What are your personal weaknesses? Where do you find it easiest to misstep? Where can you build in routine and habit to protect yourself from your worst instincts?

Imperfection

I also allow myself to be imperfect.

I personally believe in quality of life over quantity of life. It's possible I could force myself to live on soybean snacks and egg whites and get down to a size 2 (although I think I went straight from youth sizes to a size 8 back in the day), but I don't want to live a life that is bland and tasteless.

I like food. I enjoy eating. So my "diet" is never going to go to that extreme. I can't sustain that. I don't *want* that. I'd rather weigh more and live a shorter life but enjoy that life than deprive myself of all taste and experience.

Which means I have to find a balance. I needed to lose weight. (Well, technically, my doctor didn't tell me I had to lose weight. She just said that for my particular issue losing weight would help, and it did. But she didn't really expect or demand that I do so.)

But I also need to enjoy my life. I don't want to spend the next fifty years in a self-imposed Land of Blah.

And, honestly, the more you try to hold your body to something unnatural or difficult, the less likely you are to succeed long-term. There's an author I follow on social media who was anorexic for many years. One day her body just stopped letting that work, and she gained a lot of weight on a very low calorie diet.

Your body will fight you if you're trying to do something that is not natural to it.

So not only am I never going to aim to be a size 2— because that's not how I'm built—but I'm also not going to try to get an A+ in dieting.

The more your choices require unrelenting discipline and focus, the more likely you are to fail in the long run.

If you demand perfection of yourself, then losing control for a moment is a failure. That can lead to a spiral where you decide that if you can't be perfect, then what's the point, and you completely stop trying.

It also means that when you "fall off the wagon" you fall off even harder, because you've been denying yourself something that you crave. When you finally fulfill that craving there's a tendency to *really* fulfill it.

For me, I've experienced this with soda. I've completely quit once or twice in the past. But then I had one can of soda somewhere and suddenly, before I knew it, I was back to three or four cans a day. Sometimes more.

Better to just not have it at home, so I don't drink it regularly, but to let myself have one at my grandma's when I go there for lunch. Or at the office when I have to be there on occasion. Or to let myself get in a car, drive to a gas station, and buy a can when the craving is that strong.

The imperfections I allow myself are that if I go out for a meal, I order whatever I want. And the one day a week when I have to be in the office, I let myself have whatever I want for lunch. Same with going to see family. I will eat whatever they're serving.

You may have to have different imperfections. There may be too many times in your life when you're out and about to let yourself eat anything at each of those meals. But maybe you let yourself have an unhealthy drink or an unhealthy side or a dessert.

Build some slack into the system. Because the imperfect diet that you can keep with is better than the perfect diet that you can only follow for two months.

Limit Your Indulgences

Another imperfection I allow myself is the periodic indulgence, but I try to limit it at the same time.

This is a lifelong change. You have to be willing to live this way long-term. Which means that sometimes you have to let yourself indulge. But at the same time, it's good to keep it controlled.

For me, for example, I will let myself buy one serving of something "bad" when I'm at the store, or if I'm so motivated by wanting it to get dressed and go pick it up.

But I only buy that one serving. I don't let myself buy the gallon of ice cream or the case of soda. One serving meets the craving, a case or gallon creates a fail scenario where I end up eating or drinking the rest of it out of habit.

Another little trick I used to use when I was drinking soda at home, was to not have a can of soda that was cold. I only like to drink out of the can and only cold. So that kept me from mindlessly grabbing another can and drinking it. If I had to put one in the fridge or freezer and wait for it to get cold before I could drink it, I drank less. (I also sometimes exploded a can in the freezer when I forgot that I put one there…)

So figure out little tricks or rules for those areas where you want to indulge to limit the impact but still fill the craving.

Summary

As I said before, you're going to have to figure out what works for you. Look at your environment, figure out which substitutes you can make, use habits to help limit the temptation points you face, and allow yourself to indulge but in a way that only fills that craving and doesn't set you up for further unneeded indulgence.

What I do might work for you or you may need to come up with other strategies, like only ordering fish dishes when you eat out or appetizer portions instead of dinner portions. Or creating a weekly menu with a variety of healthy dishes that you follow religiously but that gives you enough variety to feel satiated.

WHAT ABOUT COUNTING CALORIES?

At its most basic, bringing in fewer calories than you burn will theoretically make you lose weight. (Assuming you haven't put your body into starvation mode.)

And counting calories does work for that. I know people who have done so over the years and lost weight. I did myself. Also, many of the popular diet programs work on some variation of that principle. Track what you eat, assign calories or points, stay below X, and voila.

The flip side of that approach is to add exercise to burn off more calories. You don't reduce what you eat, you increase how much you burn.

I don't like the monitor everything approach because when I did it, I ended up feeling very mentally unhealthy. It made me obsessive about food in a bad way. I could easily see how people become controlling around what they eat when they have to think about every meal and every action from a plus/minus point of view.

I decided that for me personally, it might work, but it was not something I wanted to continue. It had too high of a potential to lead to somewhere very bad.

If you can continue to enjoy your meals while measuring and analyzing and evaluating everything that goes into your body, then sure, it's a good strategy. But for me it wasn't. (And for many many people it isn't. Most eating disorders focus on what goes in and what goes out and what the number is on the scale and what the measurement is around the waist, etc.)

Now, I will say that it can be a good learning mechanism to do this for a short period of time.

At one point, a friend gave me a book that assigned points to different foods. I used the book to look at what I'd grabbed for breakfast that morning on my way into work. Turns out the two croissants I had bought on impulse that morning were the total amount of calories/points/whatever I was supposed to have for the *entire day*.

I had no clue. There were other things I could've chosen that would have given me as much satisfaction that would've been far better for me. I just didn't realize how bad those croissants really were.

Looking at what you eat for a week or two and highlighting the worst parts is a good place to start. But you don't want to become obsessive about it. You don't want to sit at a wedding counting calories in your head instead of enjoying yourself.

So do what works for you, but be very careful that you don't set up an unhealthy relationship with food.

And if you already have one, it may be helpful to explore that with a counselor. A lot of eating and weight conversations are really tied into family, culture, and society, and sometimes we can't unpack that on our own.

WHAT IS EATING HEALTHY?

If you're going to eat healthier, you have to know what that means.

As I mentioned in the introduction, the answer to this question is going to depend on you. If you have diabetes, you need to eat differently than someone who doesn't. If you take blood thinners or heart medications, you will need to adjust what you eat for those. A family history of gout, a personal history of kidney stones, whatever your personal concerns are, you need to adjust for them.

Which sucks, I know. Because we all want "the answer". We want to be told to do X and it will lead to Y. But that's not how it works.

You also have to know your own personal food weaknesses. Mine are sweets. For my mom and grandma, it's salt. They are more likely to binge on a bag of chips than on a bag of chocolates. I need to keep sweets out of the house, but my grandma can have a bowl full of caramels and chocolates on the table and won't touch it for weeks.

Also, what is considered healthy or not changes over time. You have to be careful not to be pulled out of position too much by those trends.

For example, for a while there people would say that a glass of red wine a night was healthy for you. If you drank in moderation and just had that one glass, they said that the other benefits of red wine were a net positive.

But now they say that you shouldn't start drinking red wine if you aren't already someone who drinks alcohol, because the negative effects of drinking alcohol don't actually outweigh the positives from drinking red wine.

Another example. For years people were told to take multivitamins, but recently there was a study that said they do nothing for you and may actually harm you.

I grew up hearing how bad eggs were for you, especially egg yolks. Now? I see advice that eating an egg can be good for you.

So you have to be careful about what advice you follow when trying to figure out what is or is not healthy. I would argue that any diet that has you remove an entire class of food is a bad diet for your average person. So a no-sugar diet. A no-carb diet. Even a no-meat diet.

Now, there are reasons people have to do that. Some of those reasons are ethical or moral, like veganism. Which is fine. But understand that a diet like that is (a) harder to follow for most people, and (b) may introduce additional issues that you need to keep an eye on.

In college I had a friend who became a vegetarian because she'd had to kill a bat at camp that summer. Fair enough. Her decision to make. But her hair started to fall out. Because what she eliminated from her diet included sources of food that gave her "essential nutrients" that her body clearly needed.

I had another friend who was vegan. Which, again,

fair enough, her choice. But that meant that when she traveled, sometimes she lived on mushrooms and potatoes because that's all she could easily find that met her criteria. But you can't just live on mushrooms and potatoes long-term. Maybe in sci-fi novels, but not here on Earth.

So be careful of adopting any diet that removes an entire category of food, because that makes it less likely to be sustainable and for it to meet your overall health needs.

What's better—in my opinion as a non-doctor, non-nutritionist—is adding good things to your diet. Don't restrict, improve.

So what is "good" when it comes to food? What should you add?

Let's walk through a couple of the well-researched, well-regarded diets and see what they have to say.

The Mediterranean Diet

The Mediterranean diet is one that gets lots of recommendations from various sources.

I had yet to see anyone say that the Mediterranean diet is a bad one, but I just went and specifically looked for negatives, because in this modern day and age you know someone out there is saying bad things about it just to drive traffic to their website.

And, sure enough, I found some websites that criticize it. Mostly because you could gain weight since some of the components are high calorie, and because it could be expensive.

But overall if you want a well-known diet that has lots of available recipes and is generally pretty tasty, it's a good place to start.

Now, what's interesting is that the Mediterranean diet isn't terribly well-defined, so let's pause for just a second and talk about searching for things on the internet.

When it comes to health information, I trust Mayo Clinic, Harvard Health, and University of Pennsylvania as starting points. So if I have some issue that my doctor told me about, such as "hypothyroid," I will search online for "hypothyroid mayo" and click on the Mayo Clinic link.

When it comes to diet, I think Harvard has some good guidance, as does Penn. So just now I searched for "mediterranean diet harvard" and that's what I'm using to tell you about the Mediterranean diet.

I also trust the U.S. government websites (they end in .gov) that talk about diseases and health, as well as the UK National Health Service website which seems to be nhs.uk, so not an official government site for whatever reason.

(I have links to those resources and more at the end of this book.)

Okay, so back to the Mediterranean diet.

First up, a pretty standard recommendation for almost any healthy diet is to eat more fruits, vegetables, whole grains, nuts, and legumes (beans, lentils, chickpeas, peas). They also recommend using extra virgin olive oil as the fat you cook with. You can have cheese and yogurt. There's a preference for more fish and poultry (chicken or turkey), and less red meat, like steak. And this one usually also includes a low to moderate amount of wine.

I've also seen recommendations that you adopt a Mediterranean style of dining, which was described as longer, more social meals. No eating in front of the TV alone. (Of course, some of us are antisocial weirdos who would prefer to eat alone, so do what causes you the least stress and unhappiness.)

The MIND Diet

This is one that I personally like. Maybe because about ten years ago I thought my mind was slipping and so I looked for a diet that would be good for brain health. I found the MIND diet and figured it was something I could follow long-term. On the first try I did not convert to the MIND diet, but adopting some of its advice was a first baby step towards being healthier.

So what does it include? I'm going to use Harvard's discussion of it, but there's also a good book on it that I read called The MIND Diet by Maggie Moon that has a lot of recipes in the back.

Under the MIND diet they recommend three servings a day of whole grains, one serving a day of a non-leafy vegetable, six servings a week of a green leafy vegetable, five servings a week of nuts, four servings a week of beans, two servings a week of berries, two servings a week of poultry (not fried), and one serving a week of fish.

They also recommend mainly using olive oil as your fat. The book I have recommends a glass of wine every day but per the Harvard website they've backed away from that recommendation now.

The MIND diet also recommends less pastries and sweets, less red meat, less cheese, less fried food, and limiting the use of butter or margarine.

Volumetrics

This is one that didn't stick for me, but I'd say that you can combine some of the concepts from it with the other diets.

For example, it talks about how to feel full so that you eat less by having soup for a lot of meals, rather than having those exact same components standalone on your plate. The idea is that the liquid in the soup will take up more space and help you stop eating sooner.

It also recommends avoiding calorie-dense foods like the fat in a steak. And eating more fiber to feel full. And avoiding alcohol since it is high calorie but not filling.

There's also a focus on fruits and vegetables.

Choosing Quality and Balance

This final one isn't so much a diet as a mindset, but the closer you can get to food in its natural state, the better off you probably are.

So a loin roast is going to be healthier than bacon. A steak is going to be healthier than lunch meat. Whole grain bread is going to be healthier than white bread. A fresh peach is going to be healthier than canned peaches. And so on and so on.

Harvard publishes a Healthy Eating Plate guide that can be a good starter for this sort of approach.

It recommends that half of your plate consist of fruit and vegetables, a fourth of your plate be whole grains, and a fourth of your plate be protein. (For protein, fish, poultry, beans, and nuts are preferred, but technically red meat and processed meat fall into that category, too.)

They also recommend that the oil you use to cook with is olive, canola, soy, corn, sunflower, peanut, etc. The key is to avoid trans fats there. And for drinks they recommend water, coffee, or tea.

The U.S. Department of Agriculture publishes something similar called My Plate.

It recommends that half of your plate be fruit and

vegetables with a focus on whole fruits and the use of a variety of vegetables. (Eat the rainbow.) It also recommends that grains be one-fourth of your meal and that you aim for at least half of your grains to be whole grains. The final fourth of your plate should be proteins and the USDA recommends a variety there as well.

It also says you can include dairy in your diet with a focus on milk, yogurt, and cheese, and low-fat or fat-free varieties.

* * *

Noticing a trend?

Of course, there's bias in the types of diets I chose to feature here. Because I'm not going to tell you about any diet that makes you eliminate an entire category of food. And I also prefer diets that allow room to personalize and don't require a relentless focus on what I eat at every meal.

I don't want to be told that on Monday I eat X and then on Tuesday I eat Y. What if I don't like X? Or Y? So I lean towards guidance that says, "Here's the general idea, you find a way forward."

That may not work for everyone. But I think you can see some pretty easy substitutes here.

For most people, they can benefit from:

- Replacing beverages with water. Fruit juice sounds healthy until you read the label. But water is just water. If you don't like water then consider tea or coffee.

- Adding vegetables. Most everyone could do with more vegetables in their diet.

- Adding whole fruit. Add an apple a day to your diet. It's a saying for a reason.

(And I once saw a nutritionist say that if they could just get people to eat carrots and an apple a day that would be a vast improvement for most people.)

- Adding a handful of nuts to each day.

  (It seems counter-intuitive because nuts are high calorie, right? But they're filling. And good for your digestion. I recently saw mention of a study where adding a handful of nuts about half an hour or an hour before a meal helped curb overeating during that meal.)

- Adding more legumes. My go-to is black beans but there are plenty of other choices out there. Eat hummus, it's good.

- Adding fish to their diet. For some it's already there, but for me for many years it wasn't. So adding in salmon or tuna is a good easy fix.

- Switching to whole grains from refined grains. I grew up on cheap white bread. But if you can switch to a whole grain variety or one of those 20+ seed varieties, that right there is a great improvement.

- Staying away from really processed foods. Eliminate bacon. (I know, it's hard.) Eliminate lunch meat, eliminate candy bars. To the extent you can, cook from ingredients rather than buy pre-packaged.

Let's actually talk about that last point—cooking at home when you're probably tired, stressed, and there's never enough money. Doesn't being healthy cost a lot and take a lot of effort? (Not so much if you don't care about shopping at Whole Foods, but let's explore that more in the next chapter.)

IT DOESN'T HAVE TO BE EXPENSIVE OR FANCY

There are lots and lots of people out there who will tell you that you need to shop the farmers' market or at Whole Foods to buy the freshest produce if you want to be healthy. They'll say you must use fresh herbs. And no canned foods. (Heaven forbid.) No frozen foods either. Just fresh, fresh, fresh, or it doesn't count.

Well, I say, fuck them.

Pardon my language if you're sensitive to such things. But a lot of life these days is about one group of people setting arbitrary rules to make themselves feel special while making others feel worse about themselves. The more you can take those people and ignore them, the better off you'll be.

Take the nay-sayers and lock them in a tiny room together in your head where you can't hear or see them. Let them "should" each other to death while we maybe improve your life a bit.

So. Let's talk canned and frozen vegetables first. Frozen vegetables can often be the best choice out there.

First, because they stay fresh for a long time. I cook for one person, and sometimes my desire to buy things at the store outweighs my ability to use them when I get home.

For example, two weeks ago I went to the store and I bought cabbage, an onion, potatoes, carrots, and mushrooms. All fresh. I also bought corn on the cob and tomatoes that were fresh.

My idea was that I would use most of those ingredients to make stir fry, but that I would use the corn and tomato to make a black bean, edamame, tomato, and corn salad. Both perfectly good ideas.

But the problem was that the black bean salad makes about six servings. By the time I as a single person ate through it (because it doesn't really freeze well), the other vegetables would have already gone bad. So that's a waste.

But you know what? Frozen corn works just as good for that salad. Canned corn does, too. If I'd bought frozen corn instead, I could've made my stir fry each meal while those other ingredients lasted, and then turned around and made my black bean salad. Only issue there might've been the tomatoes, but they tend to last longer than corn on the cob.

Now, some things you can't buy frozen. Like lettuce. But for the stuff you can? Do it. Throw that bag of frozen carrots, cauliflower, and broccoli into your stir fry. And don't worry that it won't be "as good" as the fresh stuff, because usually it's frozen when it's at a good point to be eaten.

Which leads us to the second reason to use canned and frozen vegetables. It's easier. I can buy a bag of mixed vegetables and cook it up in five minutes in the microwave, as opposed to buying fresh vegetables that all have to be prepared separately. No cutting up a head of broccoli, a head of cauliflower, and a bunch of carrots before I can eat. I just grab that bag and throw it in the microwave or wok.

Fresh vegetables (and fruit) also require more product knowledge. I know how to pick a ripe avocado and what fresh asparagus should smell like. Same with a ripe cantaloupe or cauliflower or broccoli. But with frozen or canned food, the manufacturer has already done that for you. You can just grab and go without getting home and realizing that your asparagus is slimy or that your avocado is black inside.

If all you want is to eat healthier rather than adopt "I am a healthy person" as your personality, then don't worry about buying fresh versus buying frozen or canned. Focus on getting better food into your diet however you can.

Although I would try with both frozen and canned fruit and vegetables to pay attention for added salt or sugar. It is better to choose the plain frozen vegetables over the ones with added sauce.

But if the choice is between a fast food hamburger meal or a bag of broccoli with cheese sauce, that bag of broccoli is going to very likely be better for you. At least it's still a vegetable.

Also, don't forget that dried is an option. I was eating dried apricots as a good possible source of iron, for example. But watch for additives. Cranberries seem like a great snack option until you notice that to make them palatable they add an insane amount of sugar. (Of course, try eating fresh cranberries sometime and you will understand why.) Also, I had to stop eating those dried apricots because the chemical they use on them made me cough each time I ate them.

Finally, remove that myth that eating healthier is more expensive.

I am actually saving money now that I'm eating healthier. Because things like a case of soda are not cheap. Switching from that to water has probably saved me $20 to $40 a month. Same with bacon, lunch meat, and chocolate. The more processed a food, the more expensive it generally is.

You can save even more money if you vary what fruits and vegetables you buy based on what's in season or on sale. I love asparagus and avocados but I don't eat them year-round.

Fish is expensive, I'll give you that, but not all of it. Those packaged tuna pouches are about a buck each when they go on sale, which is certainly cheaper than eating out these days. That's also cheaper than most of the pre-prepared meals that are much worse for you because of the salt and sugar that get added to make them so tasty.

And did you know that tofu is really cheap? I didn't until I finally tried it recently in a chickpea curry that was actually really yummy.

Okay, so you can do this and it doesn't have to be expensive or fancy.

Now, another thing we need to talk about: Changing your diet sometimes creates other dietary issues so you have to monitor for that.

YOU HAVE TO MONITOR YOURSELF

As I mentioned, I changed my diet this year and lost over ten percent of my body weight, which is great. Yay me. But you have to be careful when you introduce change into your diet, especially if you don't let yourself have certain foods.

If you were previously eating on instinct, it is quite possible that you were meeting your nutritional needs without consciously doing so. When you force your body into a new eating pattern, especially if you try to say "no" to certain foods, it can be easy to lose something essential in the process.

Remember my friend who went vegetarian and had her hair fall out? That's an extreme example.

For me, I had a more subtle issue. I cut back on red meat in order to eat more fish. Which you would think is generally a good thing, right? We saw those diet recommendations. They all recommend that.

But that led to low iron levels. Could they be caused by something else? Could I have an ulcer or something that's causing that? Oh, absolutely. But far more likely that it is diet-related. Cut out that nice red steak, don't replace it with the right thing, and boom, low iron levels.

What's weird is that after I started this diet change, I was suddenly craving tomatoes a lot. I added a ton of tomatoes into my diet after about a month.

That was my body trying to make up for things I'd taken away. (Maybe. It's a theory. Remember, I'm just a random person who is arrogant enough to think what I have to share with you could be helpful, but we all have our weird pet theories that are absolute nonsense.)

Even if I'm wrong on this, the point is that you shouldn't just change your diet and think, "All good now." Pay attention to your health after you make those changes and/or lose that weight.

The best approach is to go in to your doctor and get some bloodwork done before you start. That way you know your baseline and also know if you have any existing health conditions that you need to adjust for. It would be good to know, for example, that you are diabetic before you start mucking around with what you eat.

Or that you have high cholesterol. Or that your kidney function looks a bit off. Or your B-vitamin levels.

Ideally, you know where you're at going in, and then three to six months down the road, you retest to see where you are now.

Also, this is very important, you need to know which of your medications might need to be adjusted. For example, I am on a thyroid medicine, and it turns out that dropping 10% of my weight meant that I needed to adjust that medicine. Which didn't occur to me until I got tired in a way I hadn't since I was first diagnosed with thyroid issues. Sure enough, I retested and my numbers were off.

Mine was a minor issue, easily tested and fixed, but a number of years ago I knew someone who almost died when their medicine needed adjusted but wasn't. So if you're on medicines and you're going to lose weight or even just change what you eat in a substantial way, you need to keep an eye on that. Talk to your doctor if you can, and also get blood tests.

Which brings us to another point.

GET YOUR HEALTH IN ORDER FIRST

Before you make significant changes to your diet or decide to lose a lot of weight, it's a good idea to just get your general health in order.

I mentioned earlier that I take thyroid medicine. When I hit 40 I was incredibly tired. I was writing full-time at the time and I would get to two in the afternoon and just sort of feel completely exhausted. I'd end up falling asleep against my will for a couple of hours.

I didn't go in right away because I figured I was getting older, and maybe you just get tired as you get older. And I wasn't as busy as I'd been back in the day of sixty-hour weeks, so maybe I was one of those people who has to be go-go-go or they just stop.

But it turned out—when I went to the doctor for something completely different—that it was my thyroid. I needed medicine to get that back under control.

One of the side effects of thyroid issues can be weight issues. If I had tried to diet my way out of a health issue, it would not have worked. I needed a specific medicine to fix that.

If your body isn't working because of a health issue, trying to fix the health issue with what you eat instead of with the appropriate medicine isn't going to be very effective.

For some people weight gain is a product of depression or chronic stress. If you are struggling with depression, you will do far more for yourself and your weight by getting that under control than by eating a few more vegetables.

Getting rid of stressors and sleeping better will probably also do far more for you than adding an extra serving of fish into your diet once a week.

I know that for people struggling with chronic issues that probably sounds like flip advice. You're probably rolling your eyes and thinking, "Oh, yeah, sure, let me just cure my depression, thanks." Or, "Don't you think I'd have less stress in my life if I could? It's not that easy, Little Miss Privilege."

And I get that. There have been times in my life where things were just bad and there was no getting over or around it. The only choice was to get through and it was going to suck the whole time. Those were times where I didn't even have the energy to worry about whether I was being "healthy" or not. I was going to drink that fourth soda of the day and anyone who had an opinion about it could be damned.

But you're reading this book, so you must have some bandwidth to make a change in your life. If that's true, here are a few suggestions:

First, prioritize getting good sleep. Usually this sort of advice includes (1) try to stick to the same bedtime and wake-up time every day (having a dog really helps with this one for me), (2) avoid food a few hours before bedtime, (3) avoid nicotine, caffeine, and alcohol close to bedtime, (4) keep your room cool, dark, and quiet, and (5) also try to get at least six hours per night every night.

Second, if you drink alcohol a lot, reconsider.

Third, if you smoke, try to quit.

Fourth, find something that gives you joy and do it regularly. For me, music is a huge mood regulator. If I'm insanely upset, I have Cream live in concert to listen to. It burns out that intense emotion. I also used to listen to classical music when I was flying a lot, because it calmed me to have it on during takeoff and landing. There was also a study recently that showed that listening to sad music can actually boost your mood, which might explain why I like my "Bad Love Songs" playlist so much. It consists of slow country songs about bad breakups and really is emotionally soothing.

Fifth, allow yourself to feel those emotions. When I was growing up with a terminally-ill father there would be nights where I'd imagine the worst. I'd imagine being in that hospital and watching him die and then having to live my life without him. It was awful. Horrible. I'd lay there in bed absolutely sobbing. But it burned the overwhelming fear out of me so I could both sleep and function the next day without that anxiety dragging me down.

Sometimes you just have to let yourself imagine and feel the worst. Especially if you eat your feelings.

Sixth, find a way to escape for a bit. For me, I do this through reading. Even in my most stressed times of life, if I can make a little bit of time every day to read, it helps. I leave this world and these worries behind for just a bit. When I was younger, sports did this, too. When I was running up and down the basketball court during a game, I didn't have time to think about anything else.

It doesn't have to be big or involved either. Little things really can help. Pet a dog or sit in a park where laughing children are running around. Take five minutes if nothing else.

EXERCISE

Exercise will help you be healthier. (Unless you take it too far). It can help burn calories so you lose weight, but it can also just boost mood and physical resilience, too.

As we get older it's harder to do. When I was in high school there was gym and there were sports teams to play on. At my first college there were dorm sports. At my second one, the only exercise I got was moving around campus between classes because sports weren't part of that school culture.

And after college? Yikes. I had to force myself to go to the gym or to go hiking or whatever. There were no ready-made opportunities to easily be active, I had to seek them out.

It's important to do so, though, because exercise is incredibly important if you want to stay healthy long-term.

It doesn't have to be intense running on the treadmill at the gym, either. Just get outside and walk around the block. Take your time. Take your walker if you have to. Or a cane. Or one of those little collapsible seats. Go twenty feet. Or fifty. Do whatever you can do.

Or even putz around the house. Make a point of walking from one room to the next X number of times a day.

The more you exercise, the more calories you burn, so exercise can result in weight loss. (Although, depending on the exercise you choose, you may gain muscle mass which is supposed to weigh more than fat, so may even up your weight, but not in a bad way. You'll still lose inches and gain tone.)

Exercise has other benefits, too. Things get sore and stiff and run down as you get older. (Trust me, I know.) Turns out, though, that moving your joints helps them. The same as stretching your muscles helps. So every little bit you can do will make your body feel better if you haven't been exercising already.

From what I've been seeing lately, resistance training is a key thing to do as you age. That *can* be lifting weights, but there are a lot of other options out there, too. I have friends who do yoga or barre or Pilates. Tai chi is another option. I personally have little resistance bands I can use while sitting there watching TV. (I don't. This is one of my weak areas. Thankfully I have a dog who at least makes me walk a bit every day.)

Whatever you do, it's better than not doing anything.

But do watch for issues here. You do not want heat stroke. Or sunburn. Or a stress injury. I had a friend give themselves a hernia from sit ups. Don't do that.

I've also known people who were disordered in their exercise regime. By that I mean that maybe they didn't slip into anorexic or bulimic eating patterns, but they were similarly obsessive about exercising. Anything that consumes your thinking to an unhealthy degree is not good. And in the same way that some people obsess about what they're eating, there are people who obsess about exercise.

Exercise should be beneficial, not harmful. If you're hurting yourself with your exercise or it consumes your free time in an obsessive sort of way, seek help.

Also, try not to do the "I did X exercise so now I can eat Y." It creates a bad dynamic. If you want to do Y eating, just let yourself do that sometimes. You don't have to push yourself to do X before you can reward yourself with Y.

Just my opinion on that one. I am pretty much opposed to any pattern of thinking that makes someone miserable on a regular basis. Find the positives instead.

And if you hate a certain type of exercise, find something else. I like to hike and I like to walk my dog, so that's what I do. When I vacation I like to kayak or go rafting. I've also enjoyed yoga when the instructor was good.

On the other hand, thirty minutes in the gym is my personal purgatory, so it never becomes a lasting habit for me. I can do it for six months maybe, but then I fall off. Because the only way I go is out of obligation and I can't maintain that constant pressure on myself. I refuse to be that miserable.

Find what works for you. Remember this is all about sustainable change.

A THOUGHT ON INTERMITTENT FASTING

One of the recent rages in healthy-eating spaces has been this notion of intermittent fasting where you only eat for a set portion of the day and don't eat the rest of the time.

It turns out that maybe some of us do this unintentionally. When I had my last dog I would eat breakfast at about six in the morning and dinner at around four in the afternoon, which meant I was not eating for about fourteen hours of every day.

It didn't magically make me skinny, but there is something to be said for paying attention to *when* you eat food.

For example, if you eat breakfast, snack until lunch, eat lunch, snack until dinner, eat dinner, and then snack until bedtime, there are a lot of opportunities there to eat bad things. Which means you may have some easy improvements you can make.

Look at all that snacking. Is it healthy snacking? (My immediate old-school memory is of carrot sticks.) Or is it unhealthy snacking? Are you munching on candy and chips throughout the day?

If you find that you're eating unhealthy between meals but pretty healthy during meals—something that was true with me due to my sweet tooth—then limiting the hours when you eat can help. If you don't eat anything after dinner and that's normally a time when you snack on cookies or chips, that right there could be enough of a change to slowly drop some weight.

Even better if—in an attempt to distract yourself from wanting to snack after dinner—you take a walk around the neighborhood or sign up for some sort of social activity that keeps you busy. Maybe you take a pottery or yoga class. Then you have a double benefit, less snacking and socializing on top of it.

So if it helps limit those temptation moments, go for it.

But if it leads you to fight your natural rhythms, then don't do it.

I personally need to start every day with a solid base. I need breakfast and it has to be something that can fuel me through to lunch. I would be a disaster if I tried to hold off on eating food until one in the afternoon. I'd be cranky and tired and probably not very productive.

You know you best. Figure out what you need (and when) to function well, and don't let any trends or new ideas get in the way of that. But if those trends or new ideas work with the way you function, then absolutely give them a shot if you think they'll help.

MAKE IT EASY ON YOURSELF

In this modern day and age you don't have to cook as many things or prep as many things as you would have in the past. Don't be afraid to use shortcuts if they mean you eat healthier than before.

For example, I like black beans; they're a central part of my diet. But I tried cooking black beans once, and it did not work. I had a recipe for it and everything. I figured that was the healthiest way to prepare them. No preservatives, no salt, it would be perfect.

Unfortunately, black beans just cooked up without salt taste like cardboard.

The only way I like to eat black beans is to buy the canned variety that has salt. I don't even like the low sodium version. But at least I'm eating legumes, right?

It's also a helluva lot easier to microwave a can of beans than cook them from scratch, which makes me more likely to eat them if I eat from the can.

My grandma makes killer pinto beans, but it's some sort of magical process that can't be replicated easily and takes days. It involves soaking the beans overnight, and cooking them for hours while she adds various things. I think there's even a special pan involved. And copious amounts of bacon fat. It's a lot.

So you can absolutely try to cook things from scratch. (Split pea soup is very easy, for example, at least the way I do it.) But don't feel that you have to.

Don't let perfect be the enemy of good, as they say. If using a can of pinto beans means you eat at home and have legumes and don't go to a fast food restaurant and order something with tons of added sugar, that's a win. Move the needle as much as you can in the right direction. Each little bit will help.

So, where do I "cheat"?

I buy those microwavable bags of grains and rice. Sixty to ninety seconds in the microwave and boom, I have a base for a meal. It also lets me eat things like quinoa and black lentils that I wouldn't even know how to cook from scratch.

I also buy canned beans. Black, kidney, northern, pinto, you name it, I buy it in a can. I've bought the "raw" form, but they sit in my cupboard untouched for years, so clearly it's better for me to use the canned variety because I will actually eat it.

I also do this with herbs and spices. I currently have a tube of garlic in my fridge and little frozen garlic squares in my freezer. Are they as good as buying and using garlic cloves? Probably not. But I can reach into my fridge, grab that tube of garlic, squeeze some into my stir fry, and have garlic in my meal with about five seconds' worth of effort.

I recently bought basil that works the same way. Open lid, squeeze. Perfect.

(Purists will tell you it doesn't keep its taste the same way or tastes artificial or…Whatever, maybe they're right. But this is not fine dining. This is trying to eat healthy with as little effort as possible. I will say here, though, that it's a good idea when buying spices to buy quality. Don't go generic. There's a definite taste difference with spices.)

In addition to my frozen cubes of garlic, I have frozen cubes of onions and ginger, too. You just pop a little cube out of the container and boom, you have onions or garlic or ginger in your meal. Obviously those work best with something cooked longer-term like a slow cooker recipe or a soup, since they have to melt, but they're very convenient to use. And don't spoil like the fresh alternative would.

And, of course, we already discussed canned or frozen fruit and vegetables.

There are days that I make a healthy meal using canned meat, canned beans, canned tomatoes, and some frozen vegetables. Takes less than five minutes to throw everything in a pan and less than thirty to heat it up. Maybe not a perfect meal, but better than fast food and will last me three or four days.

So don't be afraid to eat healthy without eating from scratch.

SUSTAINING CHANGE

Okay, time for a hard truth. Most people who lose a significant amount of weight don't sustain that weight loss.

One reason is because your body kinda fights weight loss. It says, "Hey, we're getting less calories here, we need more," and signals a need to up your calorie intake instead of keep it low.

Another issue is that often people lose weight by doing something that is not the norm for them. It's like faking who you are to get a romantic partner. You can pull it off for a few weeks, maybe a few months even, but eventually you go back to being you. So if the diet you choose is something you view as a temporary fix, then likely the results will be temporary, too.

Sure, cut out carbs, that works. Short-term. But can you go the rest of your life without carbs? How many times do you have to consciously think about what you're eating and put a big X across things you want? The more ongoing effort you're having to put in to change what you eat, the less likely you can do that forever.

Eating healthier and exercising have to be a permanent lifestyle change.

It has to be, "I no longer default to ordering that big 20 ounce steak on the menu, but instead order the salmon." And if you look at what you're doing and think, "I hate this," you won't keep doing that year in and year out. (Or maybe you will, but who wants to be that miserable?)

Better to find things that aren't ideal that you can sustain over time, than be perfect for three months and completely fall apart after.

If I ate a basic lettuce salad with each lunch and dinner, I'd be a healthier person than I am right now. But I don't like lettuce. It just doesn't work for me. So I'm not going to stick to a long-term diet that requires eating lettuce every day.

But I do like spinach. I could probably stand to eat spinach every day. Especially if I threw it in with my beans. (Or microwaved it with cottage cheese which is really, really tasty as it turns out.)

You may be reading this and thinking, "I hate spinach." Fair enough. Ask yourself, "What can *I* sustain? What do *I* actually enjoy enough to keep doing? What fits in with my lifestyle?"

Fancy meals that require two hours of prep are probably not gonna work for most people. Almond butter, oat milk, and protein powder, also probably not going to work for most.

But some bananas? Yeah, okay. Blueberries? Sure. Apples? Can do.

* * *

There are strategies I've seen recommended for maintaining weight loss. And I want to tell you about them, but I will tell you up front that I am leery of some of these. Call it too much time spent around anorexics and bulimics when I was younger.

So I want you to pay attention to yourself if you use these strategies, and if you start to get obsessive, stop.

Unless you have some sort of life-threatening health issue that *must* be controlled, being a little overweight is probably better for you than becoming too controlled about your eating. It's a mental spiral that is unhealthy in multiple directions.

Okay. So. What strategies can you use to sustain your weight loss?

First, you can pay attention to the scale.

Now, that doesn't mean that you freak out when you gain a couple pounds. Especially if you let yourself ease up sometimes. And also if you're a woman because your weight may naturally fluctuate throughout a month.

But if you regularly weigh yourself and see that the number on the scale is steadily climbing, then you will know that you need to rein it back in. You gain a couple pounds, okay, no worries. You gain five, start to pay attention. You gain ten, time to look at what's going on and why that's happening.

(Keeping in mind that one reason it may be happening is because you were too extreme in losing the weight in the first place. In that case, you may need to let yourself gain that ten pounds to find the point that's actually sustainable for you long-term.)

Second, you can reward yourself for *maintaining* your new weight.

Remind yourself that you have lost X pounds or Y percentage of your starting body weight. Remind yourself that this is hard to sustain, but that you are doing so.

For every week or month that you stay at that target, give yourself a gold star. Buy a cute outfit. Find some other non-food-based reward for what you've accomplished.

Third (and be careful here), you can take photos of yourself over time.

If you take a photo at the start and then take a photo when you hit a milestone, and then take a photo as things start to slide, you will probably notice the difference.

But don't do this if it sends you down a spiral of despair. Only do it if it serves to keep you aware of backsliding.

Fourth, you can pay attention to your health numbers.

If your weight loss dropped your A1C or your cholesterol or your blood pressure or pulse, pay attention to that. Celebrate the improvement and note that you're staying in the better range.

We all want new and shiny. Bigger, better, faster, more. But when it comes to weight loss or being healthier, sometimes just holding position is an accomplishment in and of itself.

Also, whatever methods you use to sustain your weight loss, go easy on yourself. You're not going to be perfect. No one is. The people who make you think they are, aren't. Or if they are, they're fucking miserable. They are constantly on edge and stressed and worried about the slightest slip.

Don't be that way. Think about it like climbing a mountain. Sometimes you're going to step wrong. Maybe you slip a little. Maybe some rocks go sliding down the hill. Do you stop and turn around and go back to the bottom? No. You pay attention to the fact that maybe you're on a harder part of the trail, but you keep going, you watch where you put your feet, and maybe pay closer attention. But you don't quit just because you slipped once.

(Pushing this metaphor to the edge, you do stop, however, if you find that you can't handle the altitude or aren't prepared for the conditions. Pursuing a goal to the point of danger or when it's a threat to your health, is never a good idea.)

Also, to sustain this change, you may need to set a more realistic goal for the long-term. Aim to achieve and maintain 10% body weight loss, but be happy with 5%. I know that's not what a lot of people want to hear, but 5% is better than nothing, right?

This is a marathon. It's your whole life.

ENJOY THE JOURNEY

We're now kinda getting into self-help that requires a cheesy poster on the wall, but you need to find enjoyment in your food to make this last.

Me, I love a certain dark chocolate caramel truffle that my local grocery store sells. And there is nothing like the bite in the back of my throat from an almost-frozen can of Coke. I know that no diet is going to re-place those experiences for me.

But I also like the taste of a nice, crisp apple. And smokehouse almonds. And really good cheese. I even like cool, fresh water, believe it or not.

If every meal I sat down to was an effort in forcing myself to eat because "it's good for me" but all the while I was craving that chocolate and Coke, I'd be in real trouble.

So you need to find a way to be healthier that you can also actually enjoy.

For me that's fresh berries. Yogurt drizzled with honey. Crunchy granola. Grilled asparagus. Grilled Brussels sprouts. Garlic. A grilled cheese sandwich on really good bread. That spinach and cottage cheese mixture that's oh so tasty.

Make this something you want to do. It can't be about the end goal. If you make it about the end goal, you either are never going to get there or you're not going to stay there.

Find a way that works for you that makes you want to get up and eat this way every single day.

FIND OTHER COMFORTS

For many of us, eating food is how we comfort ourselves. It's a coping mechanism. It can be satisfying when the rest of the world isn't. A boyfriend may disappoint me, but chocolate never has. Right?

But you have to find other mood soothers. Other ways to indulge your emotions when needed. I mentioned before that some of mine are reading and music. Hiking, too. I also can sooth my emotions by hanging out with my dog or close friends.

For some people, meditation works. It lets them set aside the negative emotions that would otherwise make them reach for that decadent food.

This may take therapy. And that's okay. Do what you have to do to not reach for that hit or soothing experience from your food.

SURROUND YOURSELF WITH SUPPORT

If you have someone in your life who has made you feel like shit and that's why you're trying to be healthy, the first thing you should do is jettison that person from your life.

Changing your life significantly—which is probably what you'll have to do to move from where you are to where you want to be—is hard work. You don't need someone around who makes you associate that change with negative feelings about yourself.

Plus, that sort of person? They're just going to find something else to criticize about you.

Also, if you find that certain friends or family members are actively sabotaging your efforts, you need to create some distance there. We all have weak moments. We all get frustrated and want to give up. The person you need by your side when that happens is the person who tells you to keep going, not the one who says, "Well, you tried, now have this milkshake and you'll feel better."

There's a balance there, right. The person who is unrelentingly critical until you reach the goal is bad, too. You need to find that unicorn who supports what you're trying to do, but also supports the fact that you're human and may not get all the way to the goal or may backslide a bit, but who will still encourage you for what you do accomplish and how far you do improve.

Not easy, I know. And sometimes that's why joining a forum or meeting with a group regularly can help, because you can find those with similar goals willing to help encourage you. (But pay attention to the dynamics and make sure you aren't either finding someone who suggests toxic shortcuts that will harm you, or who isn't secretly in competition with you, or who isn't ready for you to fail so they can feel okay about their own failure.)

Life, I tell ya. People are the trickiest part of it.

OUTSIDE FACTORS

If you're doing this because society or your doctor tells you to, that's probably not going to work long-term.

At some point you'll be frustrated and tired and want to just go back to what you were doing before. If you're not doing it for you—if you're doing it for others or because of what others think about you—then that's going to make it really hard to sustain.

But doing it for yourself is tricky, too. Because the world around you will absolutely try to take something you're doing for you and make it about everyone else. You can't avoid the fact that the world will reward you for weight loss. Because it absolutely will and does.

And when you get sick of the world around you and want to assert your independence, there's no easier way to do so than to gain that weight back. "Screw you, negative person who can't accept me unless my outside meets a certain standard, I'm eating this candy bar and you can't stop me."

Another thing that's going to throw you—or at least it does me every time—is the way that the world changes when you lose weight.

First, let me say that you can find acceptance and love at any size. If you doubt me, I want you to go sit in front of a grocery store for the weekend and watch all the couples who go through there. You will learn that *anyone* can find *someone*.

But let's not be naïve here. The world is geared towards a conventional definition of attractiveness, and part of that definition is someone who is skinnier, mobile, and active. Getting healthier in your eating will very likely make you more attractive than you were before.

When you're outside of that dynamic, it can seem appealing. "Ooh, if I just lose twenty pounds, maybe that guy I always liked will like me back." And maybe he will.

But what if you lose that weight and he does? What if he finally notices you? You're the same person, but suddenly being ten pounds skinnier makes you worthy? Is his interest in you conditional on the number on the scale? Will he suddenly not think you're an amazing person if you gain the weight back? Why couldn't he see your value when you weighed a little more?

And what is up with random people being more helpful all of a sudden?

It can do a bit of a number on your head.

Also, if you're not used to being pursued as a sexual object, especially if you're a woman, it can be really uncomfortable. You were used to navigating the world with a certain level of invisibility and now it's gone.

Or you may like the attention very much and find that it changes who you thought you were. Maybe in a good way, maybe not.

Or maybe you like the attention until you find that the

interactions you have with others are incredibly hollow, because they're based on your surface appearance only.

It can be tempting at those points to want to retreat a bit. To put on a few pounds to get away from *that*. (Honestly, if that's where you land and there's no health reason driving your actions, then that's okay. You learned something about yourself and the world.)

Be prepared when that happens. If you need to keep the weight off, you're going to have to work through that and maybe even learn new ways of dealing with people that you never needed before.

SUMMING IT UP

Okay, that's about all I have to say about eating healthier and hopefully maybe losing some weight, too.

If you don't lose a pound but you manage to exercise a bit more and replace whatever bad thing you eat now with some fruits and vegetables, that's honestly a win.

Move as much in the right direction as you can and still maintain it. And make this for you, not anyone else. Who cares if they're judge-y because you didn't grow your own herbs in your windowsill? If you feel better about yourself, that's what counts.

We all have to find a good balance that works for us. Between all the various competing priorities, don't try to be perfect everywhere. Just move things in the right direction as much as you can without setting yourself up for failure.

Remember, being fancy doesn't matter, eating healthier does. Good luck with it.

I know you can do this.

RESOURCES

Health Information

Harvard Health

https://www.health.harvard.edu/topics/diet-and-weight-loss

University of Pennsylvania Health

https://www.pennmedicine.org/updates/blogs/health-and-wellness/2019/february/mediterranean-diet

Mayo Clinic

https://www.mayoclinic.org/healthy-lifestyle/nutrition-and-healthy-eating/in-depth/mediterranean-diet/art-20047801

(Scroll to the bottom of that page for more topics)

Kaiser

https://healthy.kaiserpermanente.org/health-wellness/healtharticle.simple-ways-to-get-started-with-strength-training

(This is a link to an article about strength training but they have a number of other good articles on being healthy.)

UK NHS

https://www.nhs.uk/live-well/eat-well/

USDA My Plate

https://www.myplate.gov/

Recipes

Red Cross Iron Rich Recipes

https://www.redcrossblood.org/donate-blood/dlp/iron-rich-recipes.html

Diabetic Gourmet

https://diabeticgourmet.com/

Eating Well

https://www.eatingwell.com/recipes/

Resources

American Heart Association

https://recipes.heart.org/

USDA My Plate

https://www.myplate.gov/myplate-kitchen

Kaiser

https://about.kaiserpermanente.org/health-and-wellness/recipes#

***Quick & Easy Cooking for One* by Cassie Leigh**

(Not all the recipes in the book are healthy but many are and if you're new to cooking for yourself it's a good introduction and, of course, written by yours truly.)

ABOUT THE AUTHOR

Cassie Leigh is the pen name of an author with a little too much time on her hands who likes to write about the things she knows and learns. In the case of this pen name that's raising a puppy, food, and the horrors of dating.

You can reach her at cassieleighauthor@gmail.com but are more likely to find her at mlhumphreywriter@gmail .com and online at mlhumphrey.com

* * *